Mediterranean Sweets & Veggies

A Complete Collection of Recipes to Prepare Your Daily Mediterranean Sweets & Vegetables

Alex Brawn

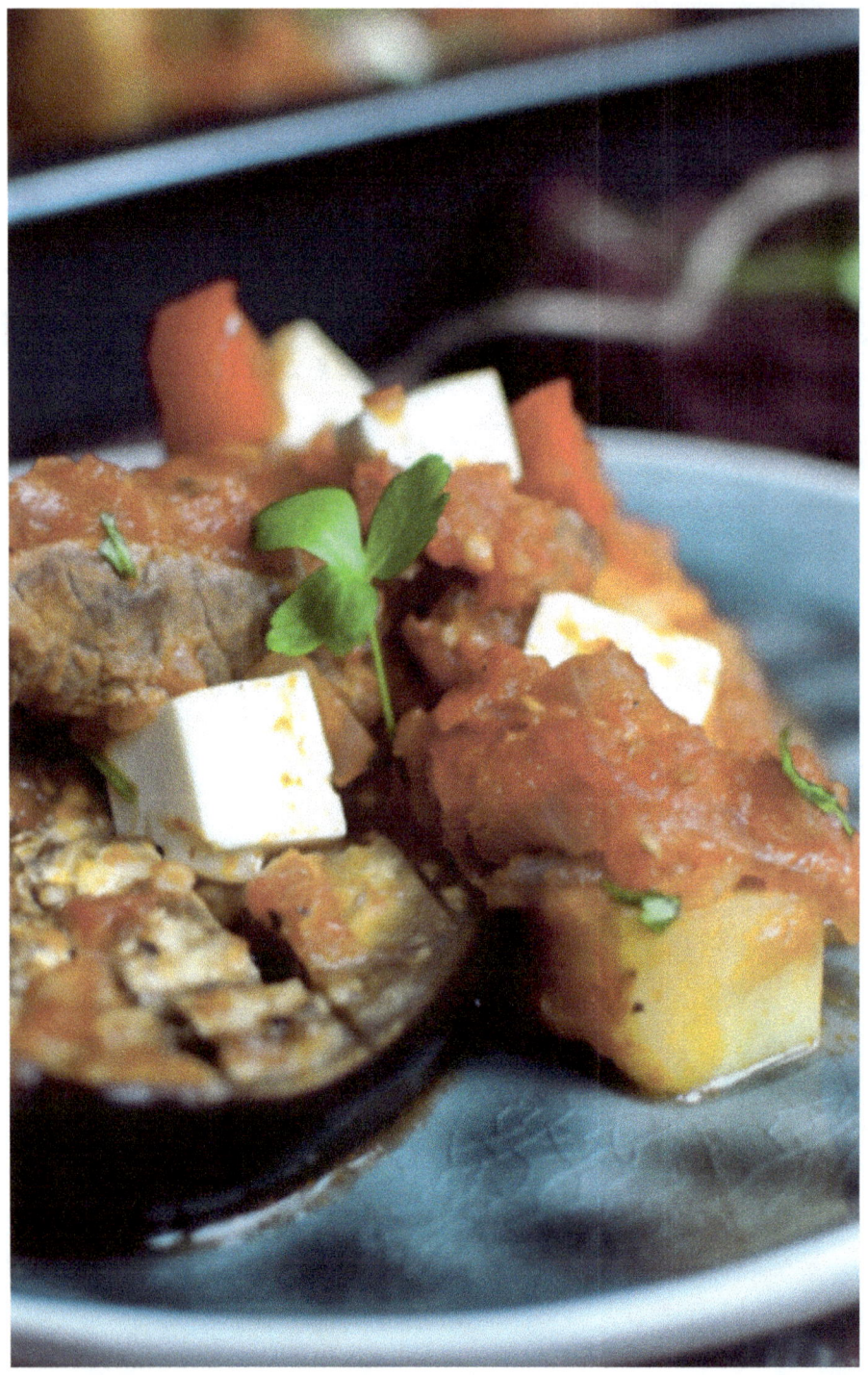

© Copyright 2021 - All rights reserved.

The content contained within this book may not be reproduced, duplicated or transmitted without direct written permission from the author or the publisher.
Under no circumstances will any blame or legal responsibility be held against the publisher, or author, for any damages, reparation, or monetary loss due to the information contained within this book. Either directly or indirectly.

Legal Notice:
This book is copyright protected. This book is only for personal use. You cannot amend, distribute, sell, use, quote or paraphrase any part, or the content within this book, without the consent of the author or publisher.

Disclaimer Notice:
Please note the information contained within this document is for educational and entertainment purposes only. All effort has been executed to present accurate, up to date, and reliable, complete information. No warranties of any kind are declared or implied. Readers acknowledge that the author is not engaging in the rendering of legal, financial, medical or professional advice. The content within this book has been derived from various sources. Please consult a licensed professional before attempting any techniques outlined in this book.

By reading this document, the reader agrees that under no circumstances is the author responsible for any losses, direct or indirect, which are incurred as a result of the use of information contained within this document, including, but not limited to, — errors, omissions, or inaccuracies.

Table of Contents

Chocolate porridge 7

Roasted stone fruit 10

Watermelon and feta salad 12

Mango chutney 13

Almond, banana, and passion fruit smoothie 16

DIY oat fruity cereal 17

Italian style Bakewell tart 19

Strawberry and cream sandwich sponge 21

Rhubarb sorbet with pistachio brittle 23

Cherry flans 25

Pina colada fro-yo 28

Plum sorbet 29

Plum lattice pie 30

Soaked pistachio and citrus cake 33

Asian style watermelon salad 35

Rainbow jelly 37

Blackberry fool 38

Baked berries with brandy mascarpone 40

Hot cross muffins 41

Poached peaches or apricots and lemon grass 43

Vegan toffee apple upside down cake 45

Pomegranate and clementine sorbet 47

Passion-berry choux buns 49

Four-grain coconut porridge with autumnal fruit 53

Stuffed fruit crumble 55

Pear and ginger pudding 56

Berry good pancakes 58

Cranberry granola 61

Passion fruit cairipinha 62

Date, cocoa and pumpkin recipe 63

Cherry clafoutis 65

Cranberry Bakewell 68

Winter ginger, pear and almond cake 71

Summer pudding 73

Raspberry burnt cream 75

Citrus poached pears 77

Limon cello and fruit salad fro-yo 78

Versatile veggie chili 79

Classic ratatouille 82

Carrot spinach juice 85

Fresh tomato juice 87

Aubergine parmigiana 88

Bubble and squeak 91

Speedy quiche tray bake 93

Roasted parsnips 95

Veggie Bolognese sauce 98

Veggie korma 100

Freezer raid springtime risotto 102

Glazed carrots 104

Brussels sprouts 106

Chocolate porridge

The chocolate porridge is a delicious Mediterranean diet drink that can keep you hooked onto it the rest of the day. The taste is elevated by the use of cocoa powder that gives it a brilliant chocolaty goodness.

Ingredients

- 1 pinch of ground cinnamon
- 3 heaped tablespoons quality cocoa powder
- 80g of fresh fruit
- 200g of blanched hazelnuts
- 2 teaspoons of vanilla extract
- 200ml of coconut water
- 1 heaped tablespoon Greek yoghurt
- 200g of Medjool dates
- 400g of porridge oats
- 1 orange

Directions

- Start by toasting the hazelnuts in a dry pan on a medium heat until golden.
- Process in a food processor.

- Add the dates to the processor with half the oats, vanilla extract, and cocoa powder.
- Pulse orange zest until fine, then stir the mixture back through the rest of the oats.
- Pour into an airtight jar, ready to use.
- Serve and enjoy with a spoonful of Greek yoghurt and 80g of fresh fruit.

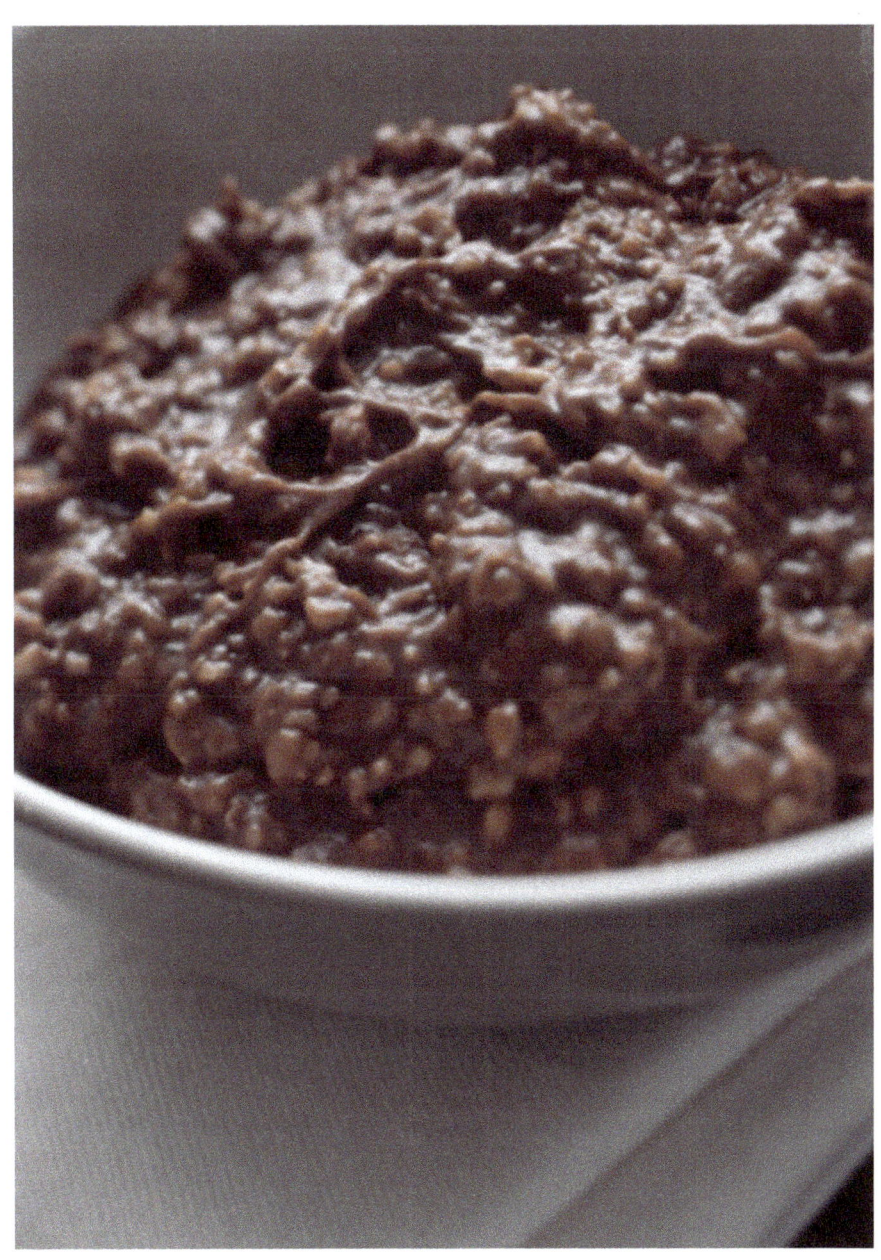

Roasted stone fruit

The roasted stone fruit Mediterranean Sea diet features ingredients rich in fiber mainly oats. This will keep you regular and eases digestions.

Ingredients

- 2kg of mixed seasonal stone fruit
- 1 tablespoon of balsamic vinegar
- 1 vanilla pod
- 80g of unsweetened desiccated coconut flakes
- 150g of ripe strawberries
- 1 tablespoon natural yoghurt
- 200g of Medjool dates
- 360g of porridge oats
- 6 oranges
- Extra virgin olive oil

Directions

- Preheat the oven ready to 400°F.
- Squeeze the lemon juice into a large roasting dish with the balsamic.
- Add the vanilla with the seeds to the dish.

- Grate in the strawberries, mix together, place into the oven to warm through.
- Place the dates in a food processor together with the oats, coconut flakes, oil and water, blend into a crumble.
- Pour into a roasting tray.
- Spread out into an even layer.
- Pull the dish of warm, juices out of the oven and gently stir in all the fruit.
- Return to the top shelf of the oven, place the crumble on the shelf underneath, and cook for 45 minutes.
- Stir the crumble occasionally.
- Serve and enjoy with a tablespoon of to each serving.

Watermelon and feta salad

Amongst fruits, watermelon is a gift to the kidney. As such, this Mediterranean Sea diet weighs heavier due to its health benefits let alone its tastiness.

Ingredients
- Extra virgin olive oil
- 180g of feta cheese
- 700g of watermelon
- 1 bunch of fresh mint
- 1 small red onion

Directions
- Chop the watermelon flesh into chunks.
- Slice the onion and crumble the feta
- Pick the mint leaves, tearing any larger ones.
- Place it all into a bowl and combine.
- Drizzle over a little oil.
- Season with black pepper to taste.
- Serve and enjoy.

Mango chutney

Fresh mango fruits are very sweet and rich in vitamin source. The recipe blends its natural sweetness with natural flavors to elevate its taste further and can be served with any curry of your choice.

Ingredients

- 1 teaspoon of coriander seeds
- 8cm piece of ginger
- 8 cardamom pods
- 2 cloves of garlic
- 1 fresh red chili
- 1 teaspoon of chili powder
- 2kg of mangos
- 500ml of white wine vinegar
- 2 teaspoons of nigella seeds
- 400g of granulated sugar
- 1 teaspoon of cumin seeds

Directions

- Prepare the mangoes and keep aside.
- Add the vinegar and sugar to a large pan over a medium heat.

- Stir to dissolve the sugar.
- Bring to a boil, let the water reduce a little bit.
- Toast the cumin together with the coriander and cardamom seeds until aromatic.
- Crush with the chili powder using a mortar.
- Add to the vinegar pan, along with the chopped mango, nigella seeds, and sea salt.
- Grate in the ginger.
- Introduce in the garlic let boil.
- Lower the heat, let simmer for 1 hour until it is thick.
- Add the chopped chili in the last 10 minutes.
- Serve and enjoy.

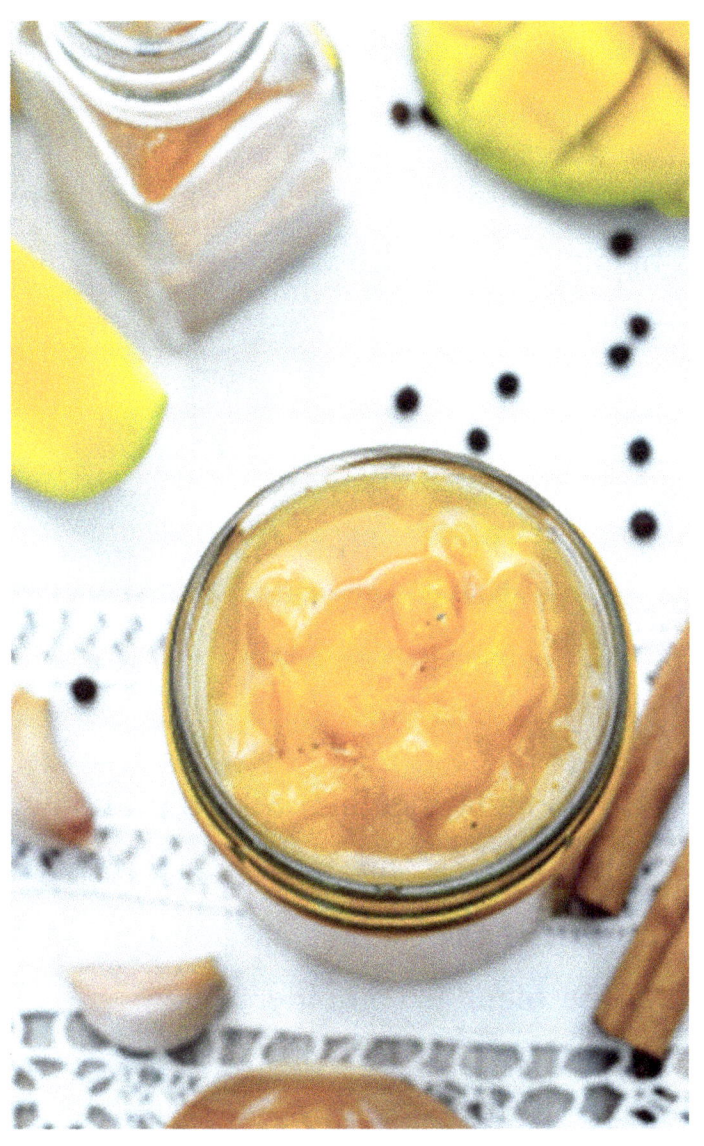

Almond, banana, and passion fruit smoothie

This is a perfect Mediterranean recipe for a tasty breakfast. It is highly fuss-free rich with variety of fruits with several health benefits.

Ingredients

- 4 ripe passion fruit
- 1 large ripe banana
- 1 teaspoon of almond essence
- 500ml of almond milk

Directions

- Place the banana together with the almond milk and almond essence in a blender.
- Scrape most of the pulp of passion fruit into the blender, blend to combine.
- Serve and enjoy with ice if desired.

DIY oat fruity cereal

Ingredients

- 1 eating apple
- 50g of mixed unsalted nuts
- Roughly 400ml of milk
- 50g of mixed seeds
- 400g of porridge oat
- 100g of dried fruit
- 1 teaspoon ground cinnamon
- Milk

Directions

- Place cereals into a large bowl together with the seeds, oats, and cinnamon.
- Place into an airtight container.
- Add milk or natural yoghurt and chopped fresh fruit, serve.
- Or, add 200g of the cereal to a large bowl.
- Place a box grater on a board, then coarsely grate the apple.
- Add to the oat cereal.
- Pour over enough milk to cover, then mix well.

- Cover the bowl with Clingfilm.
- Place in the fridge to soak overnight.
- Stir the Bircher, serve and enjoy with chopped fresh fruits.

Italian style Bakewell tart

Ingredients

- 200g of golden caster sugar
- 20g of icing sugar
- 25ml of Limon cello
- 40g of plain flour
- 500g of all-butter short crust pastry
- 30g of flaked almonds
- 200g of unsalted butter
- 750g of ripe plums
- 75g of icing sugar
- 2 sprigs of fresh rosemary
- 4 large free-range eggs
- 2 oranges
- 2 lemons
- 2 teaspoons of almond extract
- 200g of ground almonds

Directions

- Preheat the oven to 350°F.
- Place the plums in a bowl together with the rosemary leaves.

- Sprinkle with the icing sugar and marinate for 2 hours.
- Cream the butter and caster sugar together, add in the eggs beaten.
- Add in the zest from the oranges and lemons.
- Add the almond extract.
- Fold through the ground almonds and flour.
- Roll out the pastry on a floured surface.
- Let bake for 15 minutes.
- Spread the frangipane over the pastry, stud with the plums and flaked almonds.
- Bake for 30 minutes over low heat, let cool slightly.
- Mix icing ingredients until smooth.
- Drizzle over the tart.
- Serve and enjoy.

Strawberry and cream sandwich sponge

Ingredients

- 250g of fresh strawberries
- 1 teaspoon vanilla extract
- 4 large free-range eggs
- 1½ tablespoon of icing sugar
- 225g of self-rising flour
- 1 teaspoon baking powder
- 225g of unsalted butter
- 200ml of double cream
- 225g of white caster sugar
- 1 splash of milk
- 1 vanilla pod

Directions

- Preheat the oven to 400°F.
- Grease sandwich tins.
- Cream butter with the sugar in a large mixing bowl until fluffy.
- Mix in the vanilla extract.
- Beat the eggs, mix into the creamed butter and sugar.

- Sift, then fold in the flour, baking powder and ¼ of a teaspoon of sea salt.
- Stir in splash of milk to loosen the batter.
- Divide between the 2 cake tins.
- Let bake for 22 – 25 minutes.
- Let cool when ready for 5 minutes.
- Pour the cream into a large bowl, add the vanilla seeds and whisk.
- Add icing sugar and fold through.
- Spread the vanilla cream.
- Slice the strawberries, and scatter on top of the second cake.
- Dust with icing sugar.
- Serve and enjoy.

Rhubarb sorbet with pistachio brittle

Ingredients

- ½ teaspoon of matcha powder
- 800g of rhubarb
- 400g of caster sugar
- 1 lime
- vegetable oil
- 100g of shelled pistachios

Directions

- Prepare the rhubarb, place in a large bowl and bring to boil.
- Uncover, let simmer for 5 minutes.
- Transfer into a blender and purée.
- Squeeze in the juice of half the lime.
- Taste and adjust accordingly.
- Churn in an ice cream maker for about 20 minutes.
- Grease the tray with vegetable oil lined with baking paper.
- Mix the matcha powder with a little hot water.

- Pour into a small pan with the remaining caster sugar, and place on a medium-high heat.
- Boil, gently swirl.
- Let simmer for 5 minutes or until it turns to deep brownish-green.
- Roughly chop and scatter on the pistachios and sea salt.
- Let cool, then break into pieces.
- Serve and enjoy.

Cherry flans

Ingredients

- 260g of cherries
- 1 lemon
- 100g of sugar
- 2 free-range egg yolks
- 3 tablespoons kirsch
- 3 large free-range eggs
- 200ml of milk
- 3 tablespoons single cream
- 150g of sugar

Directions

- Preheat the oven to 400°F.
- Place sugar and water in a pan let boil.
- When the syrup starts to color, lower the heat and continue to cook until the caramel turns golden brown.
- Remove and divide between metal tins, swirling it around the sides.
- Place the cherries in a pan with the kirsch, 2 extra tablespoons of sugar.

- Let cook for 7 minutes over a low heat. Set aside.
- Place the milk, cream and lemon zest in a pan over a medium heat let simmer.
- Stir in the sugar until it has dissolved, when removed from heat.
- Set aside for 10 minutes to allow the flavors to infuse.
- Beat the eggs and egg yolks together in a bowl, whisk in the cooled milk mixture.
- Then, strain the liquid into a bowl, stir in the cherries.
- Pour the cherry mixture into the caramel-lined metal tins, place in a deep roasting tin.
- Add enough boiling water to the roasting tin.
- Place the tin in the preheated oven and cook 45 minutes.
- Serve and enjoy with the remaining cherry syrup.

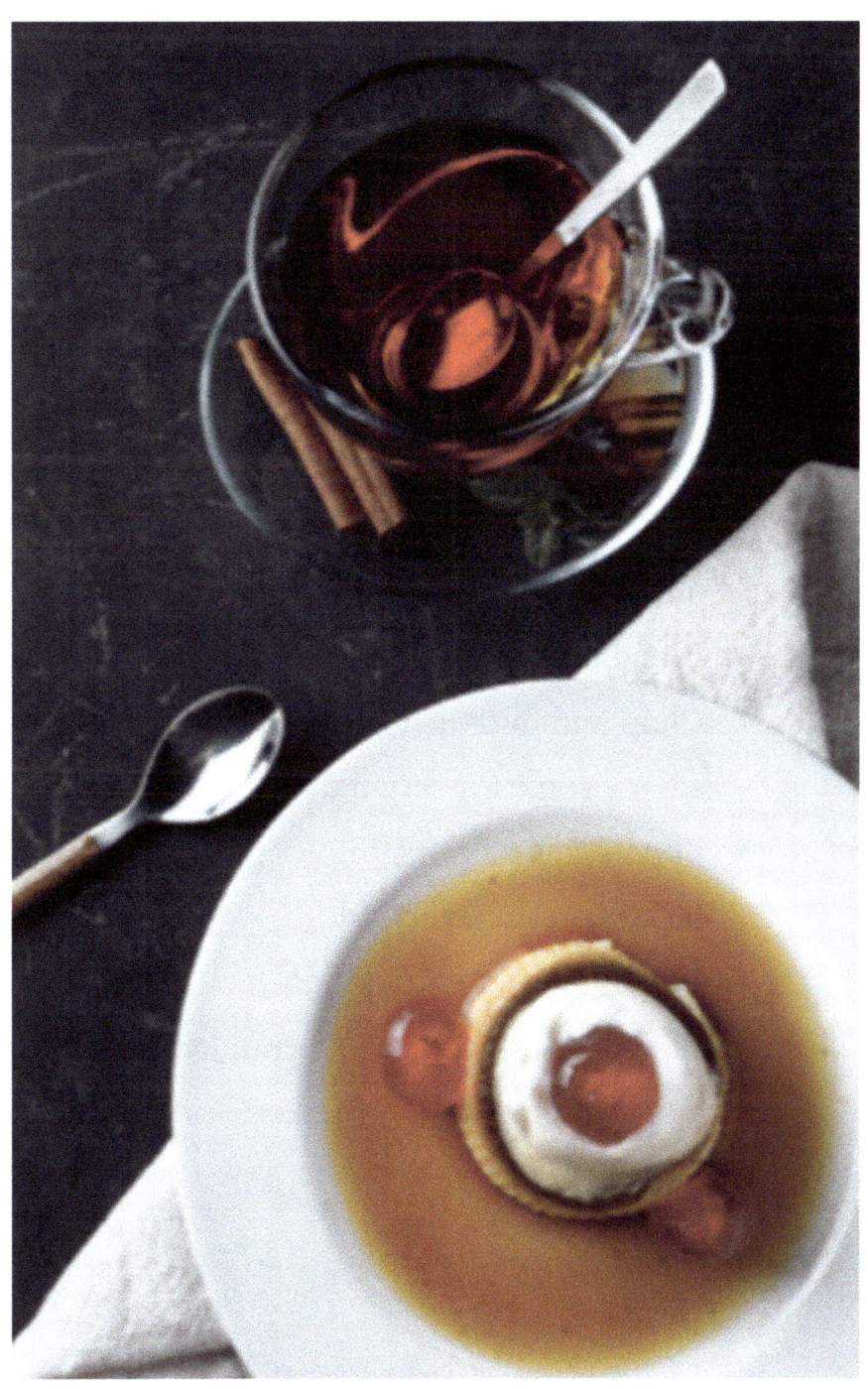

Pina colada fro-yo

Ingredients

- 6 ice cream scones
- 500g of frozen chopped tropical fruits
- 250g of Greek-style coconut yoghurt
- 75g of dried tropical fruit

Directions

- Start by adding the yoghurt and frozen fruit to a food processor.
- Blend until smooth
- Chop and fold through most of the dried fruit, saving some for serving.
- Spoon the mixture into a piping bag with a large star-shaped nozzle.
- Freeze for about 30 minutes.
- Pipe the fruity fro-yo into your ice cream cones and scatter over the reserved dried fruit.
- Serve and enjoy.

Plum sorbet

Ingredients

- 10 plums
- ½ of a lemon
- 200g of sugar
- 1 free-range egg white

Directions

- Combine the plums together with 100g of sugar in a large bowl.
- Cover tightly with Clingfilm, set over a pan of simmering water to release the plum juices for about 30 minutes.
- Sieve the plums to release the juice.
- Make a sugar syrup by dissolving the remaining sugar in 100ml of boiling water.
- Pour 100ml into the plum juice.
- Beat the egg white until frothy.
- add in the lemon juice, stir into the plum juice.
- Taste, and adjust accordingly.
- Serve and enjoy.

Plum lattice pie

Ingredients

- 3 tablespoons of corn flour
- 1 teaspoon of cinnamon
- 275g of plain flour
- 50g of butter
- 2 tablespoons of icing sugar
- ½ teaspoon of ground ginger
- 130g of butter
- 3 medium free-range egg yolks
- 100g of caster sugar
- Milk
- caster sugar
- 50g of flaked almonds
- 10 plums

Directions

- Preheat the oven to 400°F.
- Combine the flour together with the icing sugar, and a pinch of sea salt into a food processor.

- Add the butter, let blend until fine like breadcrumbs.
- Add 2 egg yolks with ice-cold water, pulse until you have a dough.
- Divide into two pieces, roll out into discs wrapping both in Clingfilm and chill in the fridge for 30 minutes.
- Roll out the larger piece of pastry and press into a pie tin let chill in the fridge.
- Roll out the remaining disc and cut out eight long, even strips, each 2.5cm wide.
- Toast the almonds in a dry frying pan until golden.
- Place all ingredients in a large bowl and stir well.
- Pile the fruit mixture into the pie base.
- Then, beat the remaining egg yolk with a splash of milk.
- Brush the edges of the pastry with it.
- Arrange, weave the pastry strips in a lattice pattern on top of the pie.

- Brush the pie with the egg wash and sprinkle with sugar.
- Chill in the fridge for 30 minutes.
- Let bake for 20 minutes, checking occasionally.
- Lower the heat to medium, let bake for 30 minutes more covered with a foil.
- Remove, sprinkle with extra sugar and let set for 3 hours.
- Serve and enjoy.

Soaked pistachio and citrus cake

Ingredients

- 1 teaspoon of dried mint
- 25g of pistachios
- 75g of unsalted butter
- 4 large free-range eggs
- 50g of no-peel orange marmalade
- 250g of sugar
- 1 lemon
- 2 lemons
- 100g of ground pistachios
- 100g of fine semolina

Directions

- Preheat your oven ready to 350°F.
- Grease and line a cake tin.
- Then, Melt butter over a low heat, set aside.
- In an electric mixer, beat the egg yolks with the sugar until creamy.
- Add the pistachios and semolina as the mixer runs, melted butter, lemon zest, marmalade, and sea salt. Blend smooth.

- In a separate bowl, whisk the egg whites.
- Fold into pistachio mixture in three additions.
- Pour the batter into the prepared tin.
- Let bake for 30 minutes.
- Combine the lemon juice with sugar in a saucepan over a medium heat until the sugar has dissolved.
- Remove, set aside.
- Pour the syrup over the cake while warm.
- Sprinkle with the dried mint, chop, scatter over the pistachios.
- Serve slices with a spoonful of Greek yoghurt when cooled completely.

Asian style watermelon salad

This Asian style watermelon salad is a refreshing recipe mainly for the summer season, but also for any other season. It features radishes, fresh mint flavors with garlic, dressing with chili hum.

Ingredients

- 2 limes
- 20g of sesame seeds
- ½ of a watermelon
- 1 tablespoon low-salt soy sauce
- 5cm piece of ginger
- 1 bunch of breakfast radishes
- 2 fresh red chilies
- ½ a bunch of fresh mint
- 1 tablespoon of sesame oil
- 1 lime
- ½ a clove of garlic

Directions

- Over a medium heat, toast the sesame seeds in a hot dry pan briefly. Set aside.
- Prepare the ginger, garlic, and chili in a jar.

- Squeeze in the lime juice.
- Then add the soy and oil, cover, shake to combine.
- Combine the watermelon together with the radishes in a bowl.
- Add over the dressing, scatter over the sliced mint, toss to combine.
- Scattering with a toasted sesame seeds and the baby mint leaves.
- Serve and enjoy, then serve with lime wedges.

Rainbow jelly

This is a veggie packed recipe with a variety of fruits with various flavors and fresh fruity juice. This will surprise your taste buds.

Ingredients

- vegetable oil
- 4 packets of jelly

Directions

- Begin by wiping inside of the jelly mold with a tiny bit of oil.
- Make jelly layer as per the packet Directions, pour into your mold.
- Refrigerate for 20 minutes.
- Crack on with the next colored jelly, pour it into your mold when the previous layer is just firm enough.
- Repeat process for all the layers and color of jelly while your mold is in the fridge.
- Serve and enjoy.

Blackberry fool

Ingredients

- 330ml of double cream
- 1 vanilla pod
- 500g of blackberries
- 1 lemon
- 200ml of fat-free Greek yoghurt
- 100g of caster sugar

Directions

- Prepare and place the vanilla in a large pan together with the berries, sugar, and lemon juice.
- Boil over a medium heat.
- Let simmer for 4 minutes or until the syrupy and the berries are soft. Set aside to cool.
- In a large bowl, whisk the cream to form peaks.
- Fold through the yogurt and swirl through the syrup.
- Layer the rest of the syrup and cream in dessert glasses

- Serve and enjoy garnished with a syrup and fresh berries.

Baked berries with brandy mascarpone

Ingredients

- 250g of mascarpone
- 100ml of brandy
- 4 tablespoons of soft dark brown sugar
- 750g of mixed berries

Directions

- Preheat your grill ready to full whack.
- In a bowl, mix the berries together with the brandy and sugar.
- Pour into a dish, dot with the mascarpone.
- Then, sprinkle over the rest of the sugar.
- Place under grill for 5 minutes.
- Serve and enjoy.

Hot cross muffins

Ingredients

- 175g of mixed dried fruit
- ¼ teaspoon of sea salt
- 225g of unsalted butter preferably at room temperature
- 3 large free-range eggs
- 50g of dried cranberries
- 100g of icing sugar
- 150g of ground almonds
- 100g of buckwheat flour
- 1 teaspoon of ground mixed spice
- 1 eating apple
- 200g of light of Muscovado sugar
- 1½ teaspoons of gluten-free baking powder
- 1 large orange

Directions

- Heat your oven ready to 380°F.
- Line two muffin trays with paper cases.
- In a large bowl, beat the butter together with sugar in an electric beater until fluffy.

- Then, combine the almonds together with the flour, mixed spice, baking powder, and salt in a bowl.
- Add on top of the creamed butter and sugar.
- Add the orange zest together with juice and the eggs to the bowl.
- Mix together until you have a thick batter.
- Stir in the dried fruit, cranberries, and apple.
- Dollop the mixture into the muffin cases.
- Let bake for 35 minutes, lower the heat to medium.
- Continue to bake for 25 minutes, until the muffins are golden.
- Let cool in the tin for 15 minutes, shift to a cooling rack.
- Mix the icing sugar with 5 teaspoons of the orange juice.
- Spoon into a piping bag with a round nozzle.
- Pipe crosses onto each muffin, then dust with extra icing sugar.
- Let settle, serve and enjoy.

Poached peaches or apricots and lemon grass

This recipe has the freshest flavor elevated with the lemon grass. It will definitely keep you wanting more for a perfect Mediterranean Sea diet.

Ingredients

- 50g of sugar
- 2 stalks of lemongrass
- 8 peaches or 12 apricots

Directions

- Prepare the lemongrass and place in a small pan.
- Heat sugar and water in the pan with the lemongrass over a medium heat to dissolve the sugar.
- Add the peaches or apricots, press a circle of greaseproof paper down on top to cover the fruit.
- Simmer gently for 5 minutes for apricot and 12 minutes for peaches.
- Cool in a bowl.

- Serve and enjoy.

Vegan toffee apple upside down cake

The topping used in this recipe mainly the apples make this meal delicious and a perfect choice for a Mediterranean Sea diet with its health benefits.

Ingredients

- 85g of shelled walnuts
- 195g of muscovado sugar
- 180g of plain flour
- 1 teaspoon of bicarbonate of soda
- 25g of vegan margarine
- 1 lemon
- 1½ teaspoons of mixed spice
- 80ml of sunflower oil
- 1 teaspoon of vinegar
- 3 dessert apples

Directions

- Grate 2 apples and slice the others.
- Melt sugar together with the margarine in a pan.
- Pour into the prepared tin.
- Top with the sliced apple in a single layer.

- Then, combine the flour together with the sugar, bicarbonate of soda, and mixed spice in a bowl.
- In another separate bowl, combine the oil together with water, vinegar, grated apple, and lemon zest.
- Thoroughly mix the dry ingredients with the wet.
- Stir in chopped walnuts.
- Pour over the layer of apples in the cake tin.
- Let bake for 30 minutes, let cool for 5 minutes.
- Serve and enjoy.

Pomegranate and clementine sorbet

Ingredient

- 5 clementine
- 1 lemon
- 500ml of fresh pomegranate juice
- 50g of granulated sugar

Directions

- Add sugar and water in a pan over a low heat.
- Stir until the sugar has dissolved, place into a jug.
- Squeeze in the clementine and lemon juice into the jug
- Add the pomegranate juice and chill in the fridge, then freeze.
- When already in ice crystals, whisk, return to the freezer.
- Repeat 4 times until you have a smooth sorbet.
- Blend in a food processor, freeze again until ready to serve.
- Enjoy.

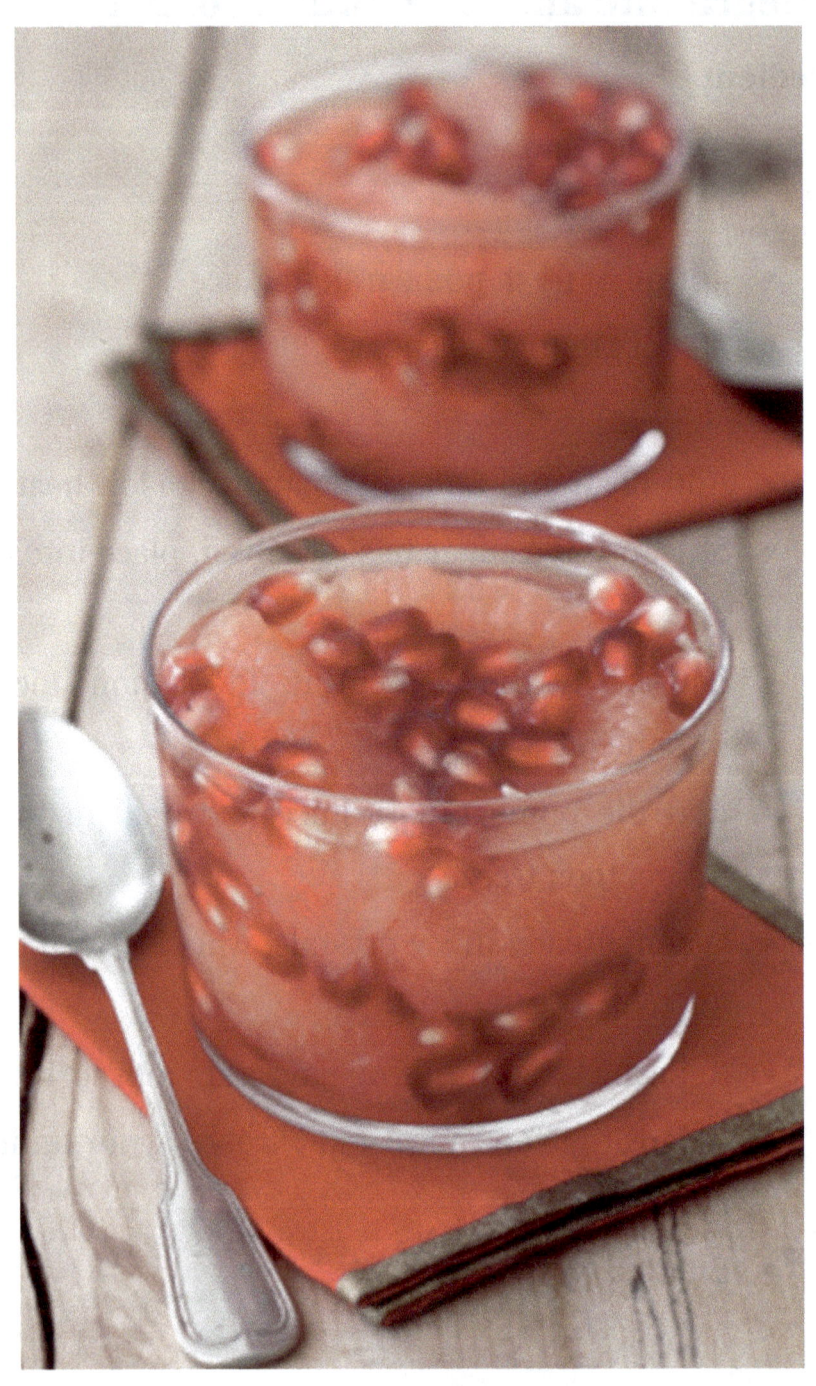

Passion-berry choux buns

The balance and aromatic flavors of the passion fruit and berries elevates the taste of this recipe beyond your imagination for a Mediterranean Sea diet.

Ingredients

- 300g of raspberries
- Caster sugar
- 1 lemon
- 25g of butter
- 4 medium free-range eggs
- 1 large free-range egg
- 3 large free-range egg yolks
- 125ml of Greek yoghurt
- ½ teaspoon of vanilla bean paste
- 125ml of double cream
- 50g of butter
- 4 large passion fruit
- 75ml of whole milk
- 250g of fondant icing sugar
- 100g of plain flour

Directions

- Place the berries into a saucepan together with 1 tablespoon of the sugar, lemon juice, and splash of water.
- Let cook for 5 minutes over a low heat sieving into a heatproof bowl.
- Mix the remaining sugar into the raspberries.
- Add the butter, over simmering water until melted.
- In another separate bowl, beat the egg and vanilla bean paste.
- Whisk in 3 tablespoons of the warm raspberry mixture to loosen, mix into the raspberry in the bowl.
- Cook over the simmering water for 10 minutes, stirring often.
- Strain the mixture into a clean bowl, cover with Clingfilm, let cool.
- Preheat your oven to 360°F.
- Dice, add butter to a pan together with milk and water.

- Place over low heat to melt the butter, raise heat to bring the mixture to a rolling boil.
- Remove pan from the hob.
- Place and beat in the flour with sugar and a pinch of sea salt until smooth.
- Dry out the mixture a little.
- Beat the eggs, add to the choux mixture, mix well.
- Line a baking tray with greaseproof paper, add choux batter onto it.
- Let bake for 20 minutes.
- Release the steam by piercing at the bottom of each burn.
- Cool on a wire rack.
- In another bowl, whip the double cream with the Greek yoghurt until it holds firm peaks.
- Fold in the raspberry curd until it holds soft peaks.
- Scoop the filling into a piping bag with a plain nozzle.
- Cut a small hole underneath each choux bun and fill with the raspberry cream.

- Scoop passion fruit pulp into a sieve set over a bowl.
- Whisk the fondant icing sugar into the juice until smooth.
- Place passion fruit icing over each bun, let set for 5 minutes.
- Serve and enjoy.

Four-grain coconut porridge with autumnal fruit

A combination of variety of grains makes this Mediterranean Sea diet recipe an energy powerhouse flavored with the coconut, you do not have to worry about your breakfast and lunch or dinner.

Ingredients

- 100g of oat bran
- 350ml of unsweetened coconut milk
- 1 orange
- Runny honey
- 10 g of oatmeal
- 1 vanilla pod
- 2 pears
- 100g of quinoa
- 1 handful of blackberries
- 1 tablespoon of hazelnuts
- 200g of porridge mix
- 1 tablespoon of chia seeds
- 200g of large porridge oats

Directions

- Combine porridge oats, oat bran, oatmeal, and quinoa in an airtight container.
- Place the porridge mix in a medium saucepan.
- Add the coconut milk, hot water, and the orange zest.
- Add vanilla pod and seeds to the pan.
- Over a medium heat, let cook for 20 minutes, stirring continuously.
- Grate the pears into a bowl, add sliced blackberries. Toss.
- Toast the hazelnuts in a dry frying pan over a medium heat, chop.
- Remove vanilla pod from the pan.
- Serve and enjoy with fruit, chia seeds, and hazelnuts.

Stuffed fruit crumble

Ingredients

- 1 large free-range egg white
- 1 orange
- ½ of a vanilla pod
- 75g of caster sugar
- 4 large plums
- 70g of desiccated coconut
- 3 cardamom pods

Directions

- Preheat your oven ready to 380°F.
- Place cardamom powder into a bowl.
- Add the vanilla flesh to bowl.
- Mix in the sugar together with the egg white, coconut, all the orange zest and half the juice.
- Place the plums cut-side up on a baking tray.
- Pile the coconut mixture into the holes
- Let bake for 18 minutes.
- Serve and enjoy with vanilla ice cream.

Pear and ginger pudding

Ingredients

- 1 ripe pear
- Golden syrup
- 1 large free-range egg
- 55g of self-rising flour
- 1 piece of stem ginger in syrup
- 55g of unsalted butter
- 55g of caster sugar
- 1 orange

Directions

- Place 2 teacups upside down on greaseproof paper, draw round them.
- Cut out the circles.
- Grease one side with butter, then grease the inside of the teacups.
- Using a food processor, process the flour together with the sugar, butter, and egg.
- Add the ginger, orange zest, pulse twice.
- Pour a small golden syrup into the base of each cup, top with half the chopped pear each.

- Divide the batter between the two cups, then lightly press a circle of paper on top, butter-side down.
- Let cook in the microwave, full power for 4 minutes.
- Let cool.
- Serve and enjoy with lashings of hot custard.

Berry good pancakes

Ingredients

- 1 handful of blueberries
- 1 cup self-rising flour
- 6 slices of streaky bacon
- 1 teaspoon baking powder
- 1 large free-range egg
- 20g of butter
- 1 cup of milk

Directions

- Crack the eggs, fill the same cup with flour.
- Add to the bowl. Toss in the baking powder.
- Fill the cup with milk, add a tiny pinch of sea salt.
- Whisk till smooth. Cover the bowl in Clingfilm and put to one side.
- Heat a non-stick frying pan, let fry until crisp.
- Put a large frying pan on a medium heat, melt the butter.
- Place the pancake batter into the pan.

- Let cook 2 minutes, until little bubbles rise up to the top. Turnover.
- Dot a handful of blueberries across the half-cooked pancakes.
- Transfer to a plate and cover with foil.
- Add the remaining butter, use all the butter.
- Serve and enjoy with the bacon.

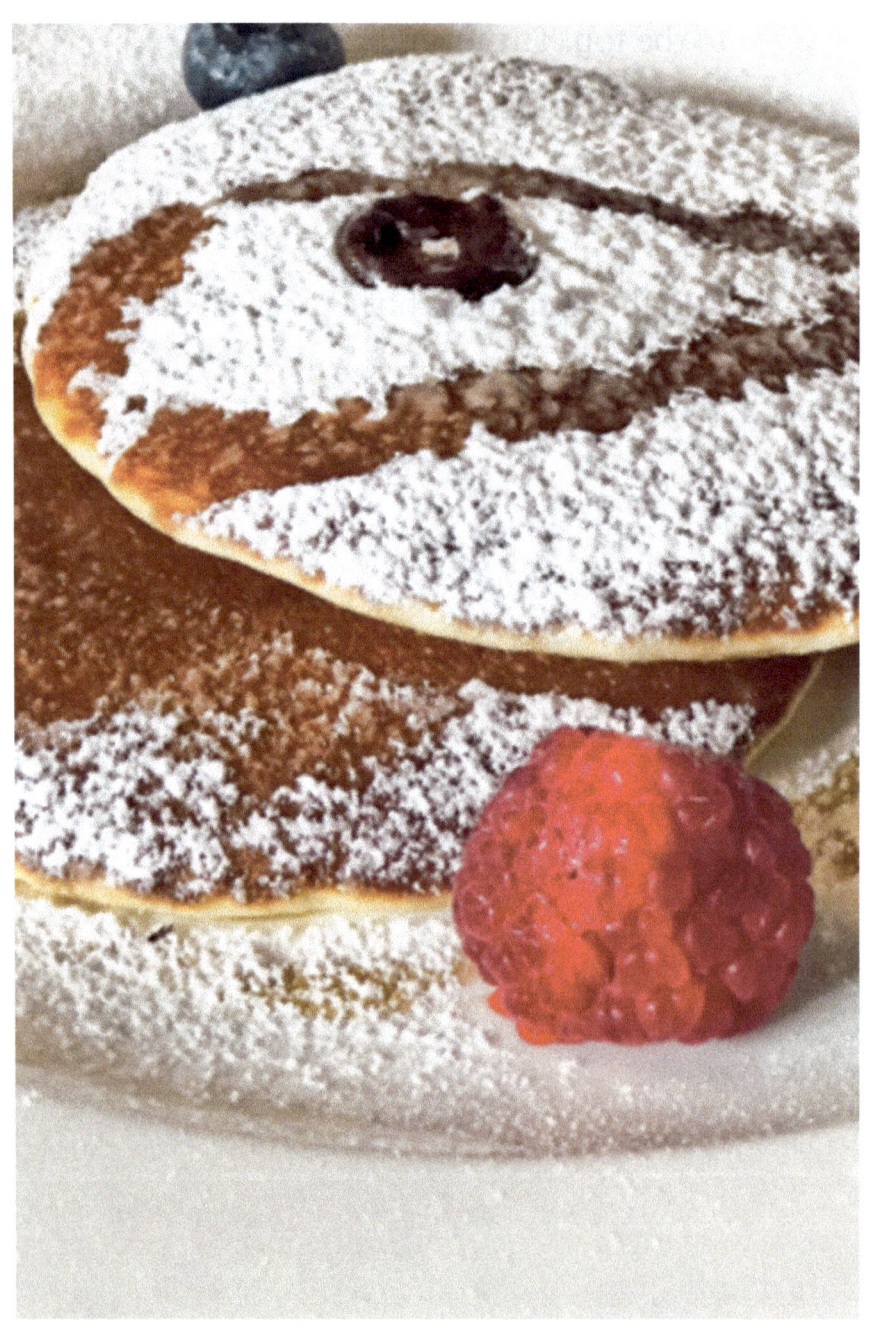

Cranberry granola

Ingredients

- 2 tablespoons of vegetable oil
- Runny honey
- 400g of jumbo rolled oats
- 100g of seeds
- 200g of mixed nuts
- 150g of dried cranberries
- 1 teaspoon of ground cinnamon
- 500g of plain yoghurt

Directions

- Begin by preheating your oven ready to 350°F.
- Mix the nuts with the oats, half the cranberries, seeds, and the oil. Stir.
- Divide between 2 baking sheets, let cook for 25 minutes till golden.
- Mix the yoghurt together with the cinnamon.
- Serve the granola with the yoghurt and a drizzle of honey.
- Enjoy.

Passion fruit cairipinha

Ingredients

- 4 tablespoons of golden caster sugar
- Crushed ice
- 3 limes
- 75ml of cachaça
- 1 ripe passion fruit

Directions

- Begin by cutting the limes into wedges.
- Place the lime wedges except 2 with sugar in a cocktail shaker.
- Muddle briefly to almost dissolve the sugar.
- Add the cachaça, spoon in most of the passion fruit pulp.
- Fill the shaker with crushed ice and shake for 1 minute.
- Pour the cocktail into 2 glasses.
- Use the 2 remaining lime wedges to garnish and the passion fruit pulp.
- Serve and enjoy.

Date, cocoa and pumpkin recipe

Ingredients

- 1 teaspoon of vanilla extract
- 1 orange
- 50g of whole almonds
- 80g of Medjool dates
- 1cm piece of fresh turmeric
- ½ teaspoon of ground cinnamon
- 20g of puffed brown rice
- 1 heaped teaspoon of quality cocoa powder
- 70g of pumpkin seeds
- ½ tablespoon of Manuka honey

Directions

- Expressly, blend 40g pumpkin seeds into a dust in a food processor.
- Add remaining pumpkin seeds with the puffed rice in the processor, almonds, and dates. Blend to chop.
- Add the ground turmeric, with cinnamon, cocoa powder, and a pinch of sea salt.
- Blend again until ground

- Add the vanilla together with the honey and half the orange juice.
- Blend briefly.
- Divide into 24 then roll into balls.
- Throw into the pumpkin seed dust.
- Shake to coat, storing them in the excess dust until needed.
- Serve and enjoy.

Cherry clafoutis

Ingredients

- 60g of sugar
- ½ tablespoon of unsalted butter
- 1 tablespoon of sugar
- ½ teaspoon of vanilla extract
- 300g of cherries
- 300ml of milk
- Icing sugar
- ½ teaspoon of baking powder
- 3 large free-range eggs
- 60g of plain flour

Directions

- Preheat the oven to 360°F.
- Combine plain four together with the baking powder, eggs, sugar, milk, and vanilla extract in a food processor, blend until smooth, keep for 30 minutes.
- Oil a round baking dish with the softened butter.
- Sprinkle over with the sugar.

- Dot the cherries around the base, place in the oven for 5 minutes.
- Remove and pour over the batter until the cherries are just covered.
- Return to the oven let bake for 35 minutes.
- Dust the clafoutis with icing sugar and serve warm.
- Enjoy.

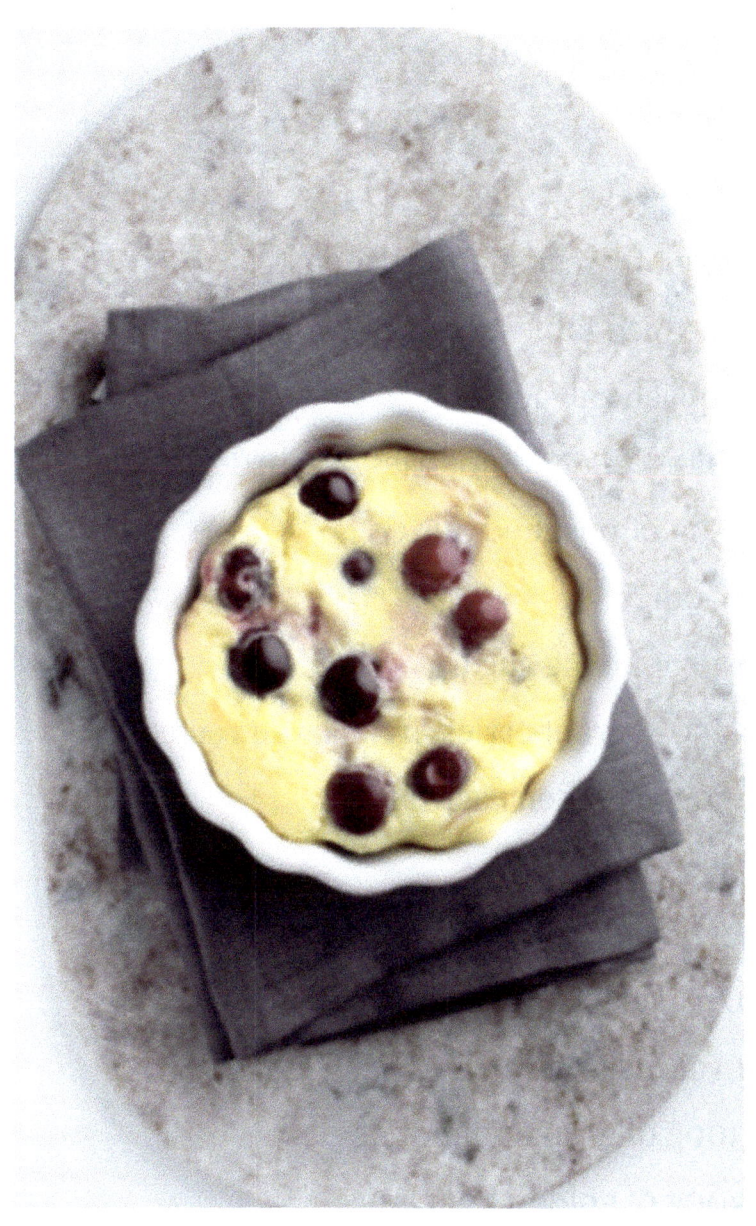

Cranberry Bakewell

Ingredients

- 2 large eggs
- 375g of sweet short crust pastry
- 2 heaped tablespoons of plain flour
- 1 splash calvados
- 1 handful of cranberries, fresh, defrosted
- 250g of unsalted butter
- 1 orange
- 100g of icing sugar
- 375g of cranberries, fresh or defrosted
- 150g of golden caster sugar
- 1-star anise
- 1 orange
- 1/2 teaspoon of ground cinnamon
- 1 vanilla pod
- 300g of ground almonds
- 300g of golden caster sugar

Directions

- Grate the orange zest into a pan.

- Squeeze in the juice, let simmer with the remaining ingredients, stirring occasionally.
- Taste, and adjust accordingly.
- Cool, then remove the star anise.
- Roll out the pastry to line oiled loose-bottomed tart tin.
- Let chill in the fridge for 1 hour.
- Combine vanilla pod, almonds, plain flour, caster sugar, eggs, unsalted butter, and processor, process until smooth.
- Wrap in Clingfilm and chill in the fridge for 30 minutes with pastry.
- Preheat the oven ready to 380°F.
- Line the pastry with greaseproof paper and fill with dried beans.
- Let bake for 10 minutes.
- Remove the beans and paper continue to bake for more 15 minutes.
- Remove.
- Then, spread the pastry with the jam, dollop over the frangipane.

- Sprinkle with the cranberries, scatter with flaked almonds.
- Bake 55 minutes.
- Let tart cool.
- Grate the orange zest into a small bowl.
- Add the icing sugar, squeeze enough orange juice to give a drizzling consistency.
- Serve and enjoy with crème fraiche.

Winter ginger, pear and almond cake

The winter ginger, pear and almond recipe is known for its aromatic ginger flavor with spicy sweet satisfying ingredients. It is an incredible Mediterranean Sea fruit recipe for a perfect breakfast choice.

Ingredients

- 20g of butter
- 220g of ground almonds
- 300g of ginger
- 4 pears
- 200g of butter
- 1 vanilla pod
- 200g of caster sugar
- 550g of caster sugar
- 4 large free-range eggs

Directions

- Preheat the oven ready to 380°F.
- Place the vanilla pod, grated ginger, and pears into a pan.
- Add 400g sugar and water let boil, simmer for briefly.

- Lower the pears into the hot liquid, simmer for 10 minutes.
- Remove the pears from the liquid let cool.
- Line a cake tin with greaseproof paper.
- Combine the remaining 150g sugar and water in a pan over a high heat.
- Simmer for 15 minutes until dark golden brown.
- Stir in the butter until you get a caramel, then pour into cake tin.
- Slices cooled pears, arrange in the warm caramel.
- Mix butter with sugar until smooth.
- Add the eggs one at a time, mix well one after the other.
- Add the almonds and mix to combine.
- Pour the cake mixture over the pears let bake 35 minutes in the heated oven.
- Serve and enjoy.

Summer pudding

Ingredients

- 2 tablespoons of red berry jam
- 150g of sugar
- ½ of an orange
- ½ teaspoon of vanilla paste
- 800g of mixed summer berries
- Olive oil
- 7 large slices of white bread

Directions

- Grease a pudding basin with oil.
- Align with 2 sheets of Clingfilm.
- Place the berries in a large saucepan together with the sugar, orange juice, and vanilla paste.
- Over low heat, let cook for 5 minutes or till the juices start bleeding from the fruit. Let cool.
- Remove the crusts from the bread, spread over the jam.
- Line the basin with 6 of the slices, jam-side up with no gaps.
- Press the bread against the sides.

- Spoon the cooled fruit and pour its juice into the lined basin, reserving some.
- Cover the pudding with the last slice of bread, jam-side down.
- Place a saucer that fits inside the basin on top of the pudding, then place a weight, on top.
- Refrigerate 12 hours to soak the juices.
- Strain the leftover juice through a fine sieve into a small pan.
- Let boil, simmer for 10 minutes.
- Drizzle large slices with the syrup.
- Serve and enjoy with crème fraiche.

Raspberry burnt cream

Ingredients

- 100g of raspberries
- 150ml of double cream
- 4 large free-range egg yolks
- 1 vanilla pod
- 2 tablespoons of golden caster sugar
- 150ml of single cream

Directions

- Preheat the oven to 300°F.
- Add vanilla pod to a pan with the creams over a low heat.
- In a bowl, whisk the egg yolks with sugar.
- Add in the hot cream, whisk frequently to make a custard.
- Strain through a sieve into a jug.
- Boil water.
- Divide the berries between four small ovenproof ramekins, then fill each with the custard.

- Place ramekins in roasting tray, pour in hot water halfway up the sides.
- Let cook in the oven for 20 minutes.
- Remove, let cool, then cover each ramekin with Clingfilm, refrigerate overnight.
- Sprinkle sugar over the custards, burn the top with a blowtorch.
- Allow to stand to let the burnt sugar hardens, then return to the fridge and chill until needed.
- Enjoy.

Citrus poached pears

Ingredients

- Double cream
- 1 lemon
- 2 pears
- 1 stick of cinnamon
- 200g of granulated sugar
- 1 orange

Directions

- Place the peeled zest and juice from the lemon, orange into a saucepan.
- Add the cinnamon together with the sugar, add 500ml of water and bring to the boil, until the sugar dissolves.
- Add the pears into the syrup once the sugar has dissolved.
- Let simmer 12 minutes or until tender.
- Remove and let cool.
- Serve the pears with double cream and or with 4 tablespoons of poaching.
- Enjoy.

Limon cello and fruit salad fro-yo

Ingredients

- 75ml of Limon cello
- 1kg of chopped mixed fruit
- Ice-cream cones
- 250ml of fat-free natural yoghurt
- Runny honey

Directions

- Blend the fruit together with the yoghurt, 2 tablespoons of honey, and the limon cello in a food processor until smooth.
- Taste and adjust accordingly.
- Spoon into a dish and freeze for 2 hours, until frozen.
- Remove and place back into the processor, blend again to break up any ice crystals. Enjoy.

Versatile veggie chili

The versatile veggie chili recipe is quite delicious and a hearty substitution to traditional chili. It features butternut squash, leek and spring onions for a greater flavor coupled with cayenne pepper for a perfect choice of a Mediterranean Sea diet.

Ingredients

- 1 heaped teaspoon ground cumin
- Lime or lemon juice, or vinegar
- Olive oil
- 2 mixed-color peppers
- 2 cloves of garlic
- 1 level teaspoon cayenne pepper
- 2 x 400g of tins of beans
- 1 bunch of fresh coriander
- 2 fresh mixed-color chilies
- 1 onion
- 1 level teaspoon ground cinnamon
- 2 x 400g of tins of quality plum tomatoes
- 500g of sweet potatoes

Directions

- Preheat the oven ready to 400°F.
- Prepare and place chopped potatoes onto a baking tray.
- Sprinkle with a pinch of cayenne, cinnamon, cumin, sea salt and black pepper.
- Drizzle with oil then toss to coat.
- Let roast for 1 hour or until golden.
- Place 2 tablespoons of oil in a large pan over a medium-high heat.
- Add the onion together with peppers, and garlic.
- Let cook for 5 minutes, stirring regularly.
- Add the coriander stalks together with the chilies and spices.
- Cook for more 10 minutes or until softened, stirring occasionally.
- Add the beans, juice and all.
- Tip in the tomatoes, breaking them up with the back of a spoon, stir well.
- Let boil, lower the heat to medium-low for 30 minutes.

- Stir the roasted sweet potato through the chili with most of the coriander leaves,
- Taste and adjust accordingly.
- Add a squeeze of lime or lemon juice or a swig of vinegar.
- Serve and enjoy with yogurt or sour cream.

Classic ratatouille

Ingredients

- 2 red onions
- 4 cloves of garlic
- 2 aborigines
- 3 courgettes
- 3 red or yellow peppers
- 6 ripe tomatoes
- ½ a bunch of fresh basil
- Olive oil
- A few sprigs of fresh thyme
- 1 x 400 g tin of quality plum tomatoes
- 1 tablespoon of balsamic vinegar
- ½ of a lemon

Directions

- Start by heating 2 tablespoons of oil in a large casserole pan over a medium heat.
- Add the chopped aubergines together with the courgettes and peppers.
- Let fry for 5 minutes, spoon the cooked vegetables into a large bowl.

- Add the onion, garlic, basil stalks, and thyme leaves with another drizzle of oil to the pan.
- Let fry for 15 minutes or until golden.
- Return the cooked veggie to the pan.
- Stir in the fresh and tinned tomatoes together with the balsamic and a pinch of sea salt and black pepper.
- Cover and let simmer over a low heat for 35 minutes.
- Tear in the basil leaves, grate in the lemon zest.
- Taste and adjust seasoning accordingly.
- Serve and enjoy with steamed rice.

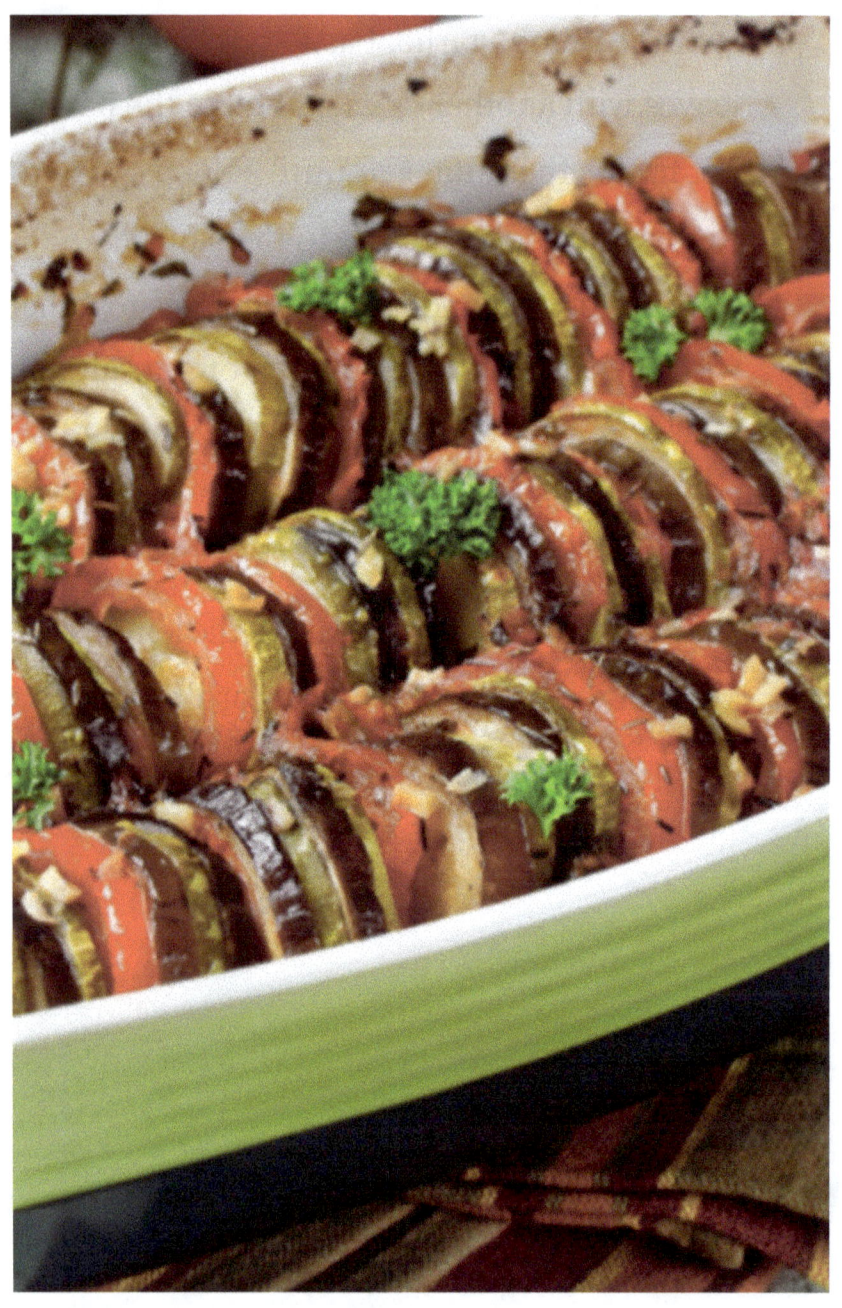

Carrot spinach juice

Combining carrots with spinach provides a rich source of iron, calcium, and vitamins along with other mineral. It is a tastier Mediterranean juice with a simple step-by-step method.

Ingredients

- 6 medium size carrots
- 1 large bunch of spinach
- Celery stalk
- ½ of lemon
- 1 ½ cups of water

Directions

- Combine the carrots together with the celery stalk and all the water in a blender.
- Blend to puree.
- Then, add the spinach and juice of lemon, (squeeze).
- Blend briefly, then, strain.
- Serve and enjoy.

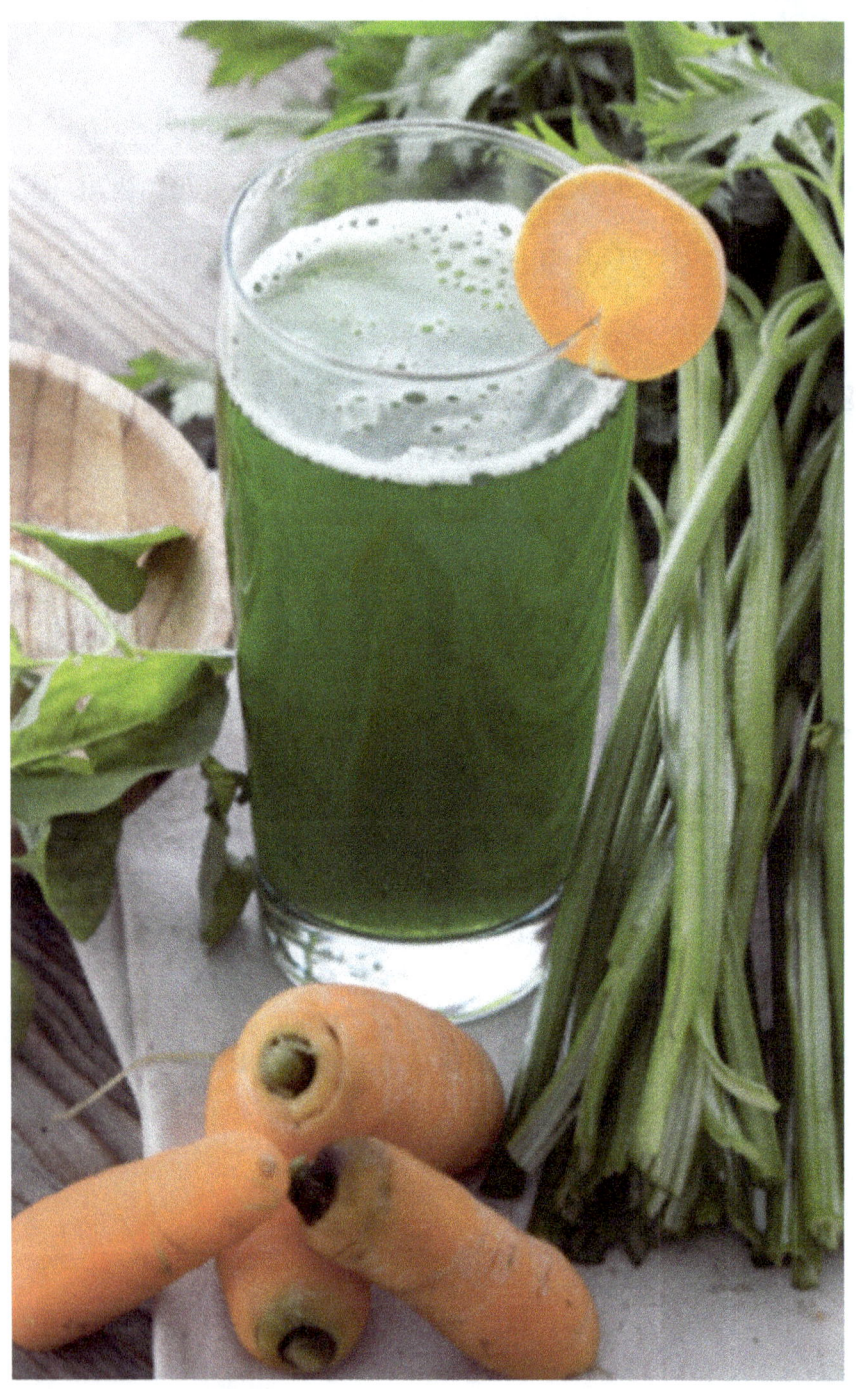

Fresh tomato juice

Ingredients

- Celery stalks
- Salt
- 2 ice cubes
- ¼ teaspoon of ground black pepper
- 2 carrots
- 6 ripe tomatoes

Directions

- Place tomatoes together with the carrots and celery in a blender.
- Blend until smooth.
- Then, add salt with black pepper to season, mix well.
- Add the ice cubes in serving glasses.
- Serve and enjoy.

Aubergine parmigiana

This a great meal recipe originating from the parts of northern Italy making a perfect Mediterranean Sea diet with variety of vegetables. It can be served perfectly with roasted fish.

Ingredients

- 1 bunch of fresh basil
- A few sprigs of fresh oregano
- 3 large firm aubergines
- 2 handfuls of dried breadcrumbs
- 150g of buffalo mozzarella
- Olive oil
- ½ a bulb of spring garlic
- 1 heaped teaspoon dried oregano
- 2 x 400g tins of quality plum tomatoes
- Wine vinegar
- 1 onion
- 3 large handfuls of parmesan cheese

Directions

- Preheat a griddle barbecue ready.

- Place a large pan on a medium heat with olive oil.
- Add the onion together with the garlic and dried oregano.
- Let cook for 10 minutes.
- Add the tomato flesh to onion pan, stir well, cover and let simmer 15 minutes over low heat.
- Grill the aubergines on both sides until lightly charred.
- Season the tomato sauce with sea salt, black pepper and a tiny swig of wine vinegar.
- Pick in the basil.
- Spoon a layer of tomato sauce into a baking dish.
- Add a scattering of Parmesan, then single layer of aubergines.
- Repeat these layers until all the ingredients are used.
- Toss chopped oregano with breadcrumbs and some olive oil.
- Sprinkle on top of the Parmesan.
- Tear over the mozzarella.

- Let bake 30 minutes.
- Serve and enjoy.

Bubble and squeak

Ingredients

- 600g of leftover cooked vegetables.
- 600g of leftover roast potatoes
- olive oil
- leftover vac-packed shell nuts
- 25g of unsalted butter
- 4 sprigs of fresh woody herbs

Directions

- Place a non-stick frying pan on a medium heat with little olive oil and butter.
- Pick in the fresh herb leaves, let crisp up briefly.
- Add the potatoes, vegetables, and any leftover shell nuts.
- Season with sea salt and black pepper.
- Let cook for 4 minutes or until golden crust forms on the bottom.
- Using a fish slice, fold crispy bits back into the mash.

- Let crisp up again, then repeat the process for 20 minutes.
- Taste and adjust the seasoning accordingly.
- Serve and enjoy with fried eggs and or lemon-dressed watercress.

Speedy quiche tray bake

Ingredients

- 6 medium free-range eggs
- 1 x 250g pack of ready-rolled filo pastry
- 55g of mature Cheddar cheese
- 1 large courgette
- 1 bunch of spring onions
- Olive oil
- 300g of broccoli

Directions

- Start by preheating the oven ready to 350°F.
- Then, grease a large roasting tray with bit of olive oil.
- Crack the eggs into a bowl and beat well.
- Layer the filo sheets into the tray, laying one sheet horizontally, and the next vertically, repeating as you layer.
- Bush with bit of egg between each sheet.
- Add a final brush to the last layer and scrunch up any excess pastry.

- Add slice spring onions, cheddar cheese, courgette, and broccoli to the bowl.
- Season with sea salt and black pepper, mix.
- Pour the mixture into the prepared pastry case, spreading out.
- Sprinkle the remaining cheese over the top.
- Let cook for 35 minutes, until the pastry is golden.
- Serve and enjoy.

Roasted parsnips

This recipe is infused with the acidity of the vinegar that strikes through the entire recipe with bay and honey.

Ingredients

- 4 fresh bay leaves
- 2 tablespoons of runny honey
- 1.5kg of medium parsnips
- 1 tablespoon of white or red wine vinegar
- 50g of unsalted butter

Ingredients

- Firstly, preheat your oven ready to 350°F.
- Blanch whole in a large pan of boiling salted water for 5 minutes.
- Drain off the water and steam dry.
- Tip into a large roasting tray.
- Dot over the butter and a pinch of sea salt and black pepper, toss to coat.
- Organize in a single layer, let roast for at least 1 hour.
- Remove from oven, quickly scatter over the bay leaves.

- Drizzle with the vinegar and honey, toss together.
- Continue to roast for 10 minutes or until golden.
- Serve and enjoy.

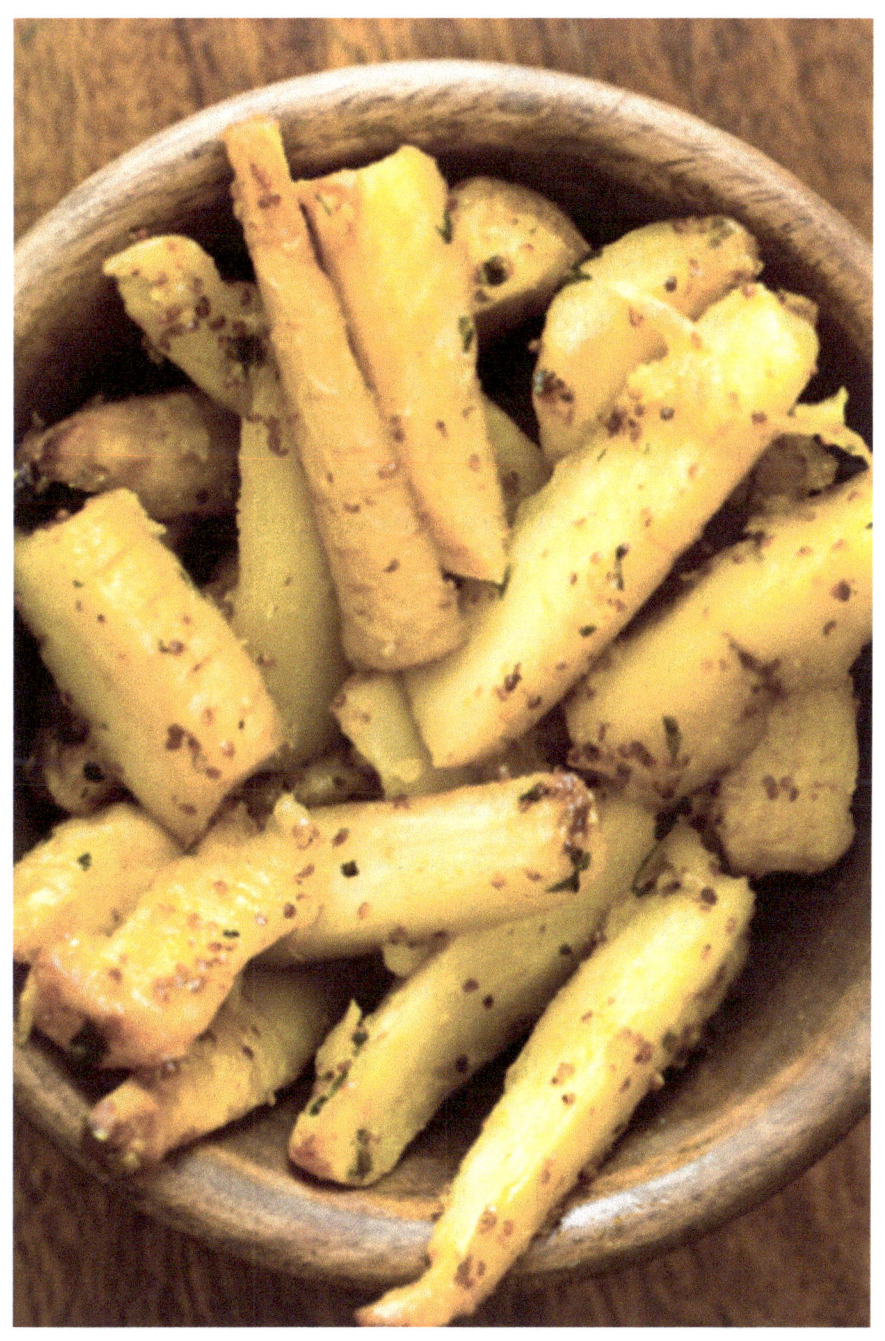

Veggie Bolognese sauce

Ingredients

- 250g of alliums
- 1 liter tomato base sauce
- 12g of garlic
- 1 tablespoon of dried mixed herbs
- 1 veggie stock cube
- 750g of Mediterranean veggies
- 25ml of olive oil
- 250g of lentils

Directions

- Place a large pan to hold all the ingredients on a medium heat with the olive oil.
- Add the alliums together with the garlic.
- Let cook for 20 minutes.
- Add the chopped Mediterranean vegetables with the herbs.
- Let cook for 15 minutes or until the vegetables are golden.
- Crush the vegetables.

- Add the lentils with the tomato base sauce, boil.
- Add water and stock cube stir well.
- Boil, lower the heat, let simmer for 40 minutes.
- Season with sea salt and black pepper.
- Serve and enjoy.

Veggie korma

Ingredients

- 2 x 400g tins of chickpeas
- 500g of alliums
- lemon juice
- 175g of plain yoghurt
- 350ml of white base sauce
- 30ml of olive oil
- 2 tablespoons of curry powder
- 2 teaspoons of smoked paprika
- 1kg of mixed vegetables
- 750ml of curry base sauce

Directions

- Place all the ingredients in large a pan over medium heat with the oil.
- Add the alliums together with the curry powder and smoked paprika.
- Cook until the alliums are golden in 20 minutes stirring frequently.
- Add chopped vegetables apart form leafy greens, to the pan, cover let cook briefly.

- Pour in the curry and white sauces with the chickpeas and water.
- Bring to the boil, lower the heat let simmer for 35 minutes.
- Add the reserved leafy vegetables.
- Boil again, let cook until the curry has reduced.
- Stir in the yoghurt until warmed through.
- Season with lemon juice, salt and black pepper.
- Serve and enjoy.

Freezer raid springtime risotto

Ingredients

- 300g of mixed frozen green vegetables
- 1 liter of vegetable stock
- Extra virgin olive oil
- 1 onion
- 1 stick of celery
- 60g of freshly grated parmesan cheese
- 1 lemon
- Olive oil
- 2 knobs of unsalted butter
- 300g of risotto rice
- 125ml of white wine

Directions

- Simmer the stock in a pan over a low heat.
- Place 1 tablespoon of olive oil together with knob of butter, onion, and celery into a pan over low heat.
- Season lightly with sea salt and black pepper.
- Cook for 10 minutes, stirring occasionally, until the vegetables are soft.

- Increase the heat to medium.
- Add the rice and stir for 2 minutes, pour in the wine and stir to absorb.
- Add hot stock, stir until fully absorbed, then add more.
- Cook for 18 minutes, adding more stock every minute, stirring regularly.
- Stir in the frozen veggies to cook through 5 minutes to rice cook time.
- Stir in the remaining butter and the Parmesan, season accordingly when heat is off.
- Drizzle with extra virgin olive oil, squeeze in bit of lemon juice per portion.
- Enjoy.

Glazed carrots

Ingredients

- 50g of unsalted butter
- 2 fresh bay leaves
- 1 tablespoon of dripping
- 2 clementine
- 2 tablespoons of runny honey
- 1kg of small mixed-color carrots
- 6 cloves of garlic
- 8 sprigs of fresh thyme

Directions

- Melt the butter in a large frying pan over a medium heat.
- Add crushed garlic to the pan, turn frequently.
- Sprinkle in the thyme sprigs, clementine juice and honey, bay, and a splash of water.
- Add the carrots, sprinkle with sea salt and black pepper, shake to coat.
- Cover, lower heat to medium-low let cook for 15 minutes.
- Serve and enjoy.

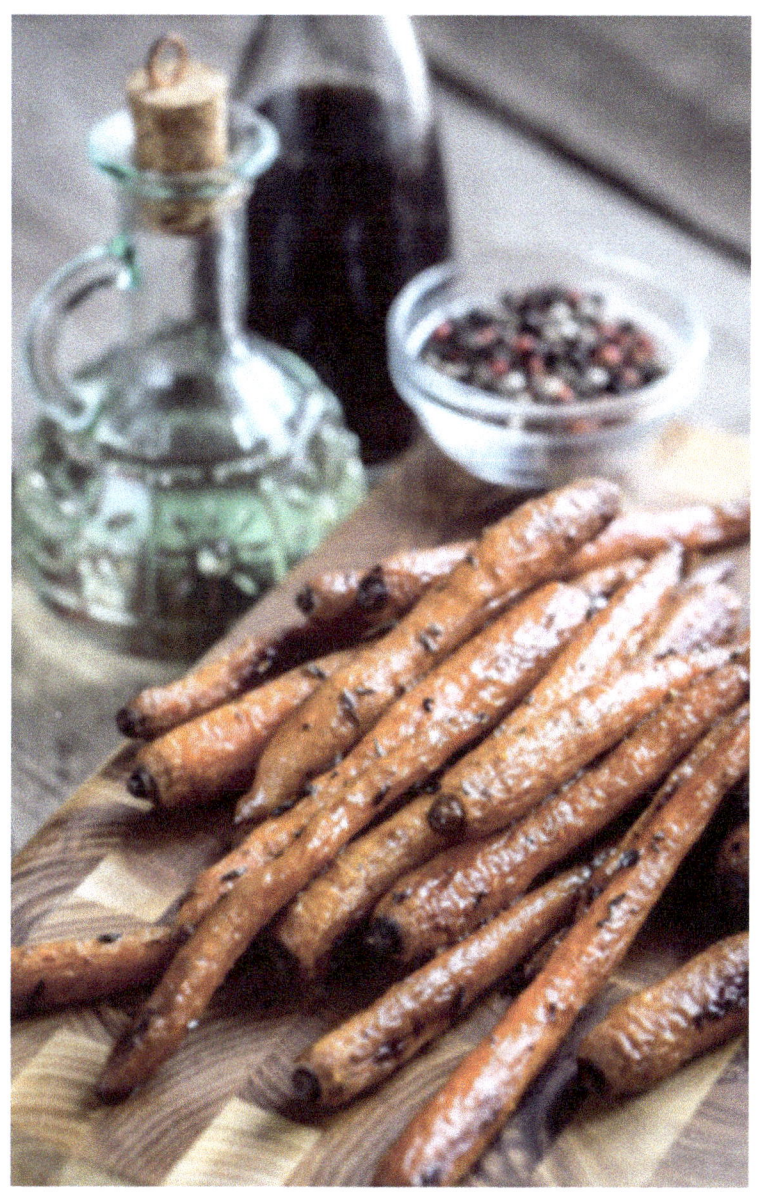

Brussels sprouts

The Brussels sprouts are insanely delicious with apple cubes, Worcestershire and sausages for a great Mediterranean Sea diet.

Ingredients

- 1 sweet eating apple
- 1 tablespoon of Worcestershire sauce
- 2 higher-welfare Cumberland sausages
- 1 onion
- 800g of Brussels sprouts
- ½ a bunch of fresh sage
- 20g of unsalted butter

Directions

- Cook the Brussels in a large pan of boiling salted water for 5 minutes.
- Drain any excess water, let steam dry.
- Melt butter in a large frying pan on a medium-low heat.
- Add half the sage leaves and let cook for 3 minutes, transfer into a small bowl.

- Place the pan back on the heat, add the sausage to the pan.
- Cook for 5 minutes, until golden.
- Add the onion with the chopped sage let cook for 5 minutes over medium heat, stirring occasionally.
- Add sliced apples with sprouts, Worcestershire sauce and toss.
- Serve and enjoy with scatter sage leaves on top.

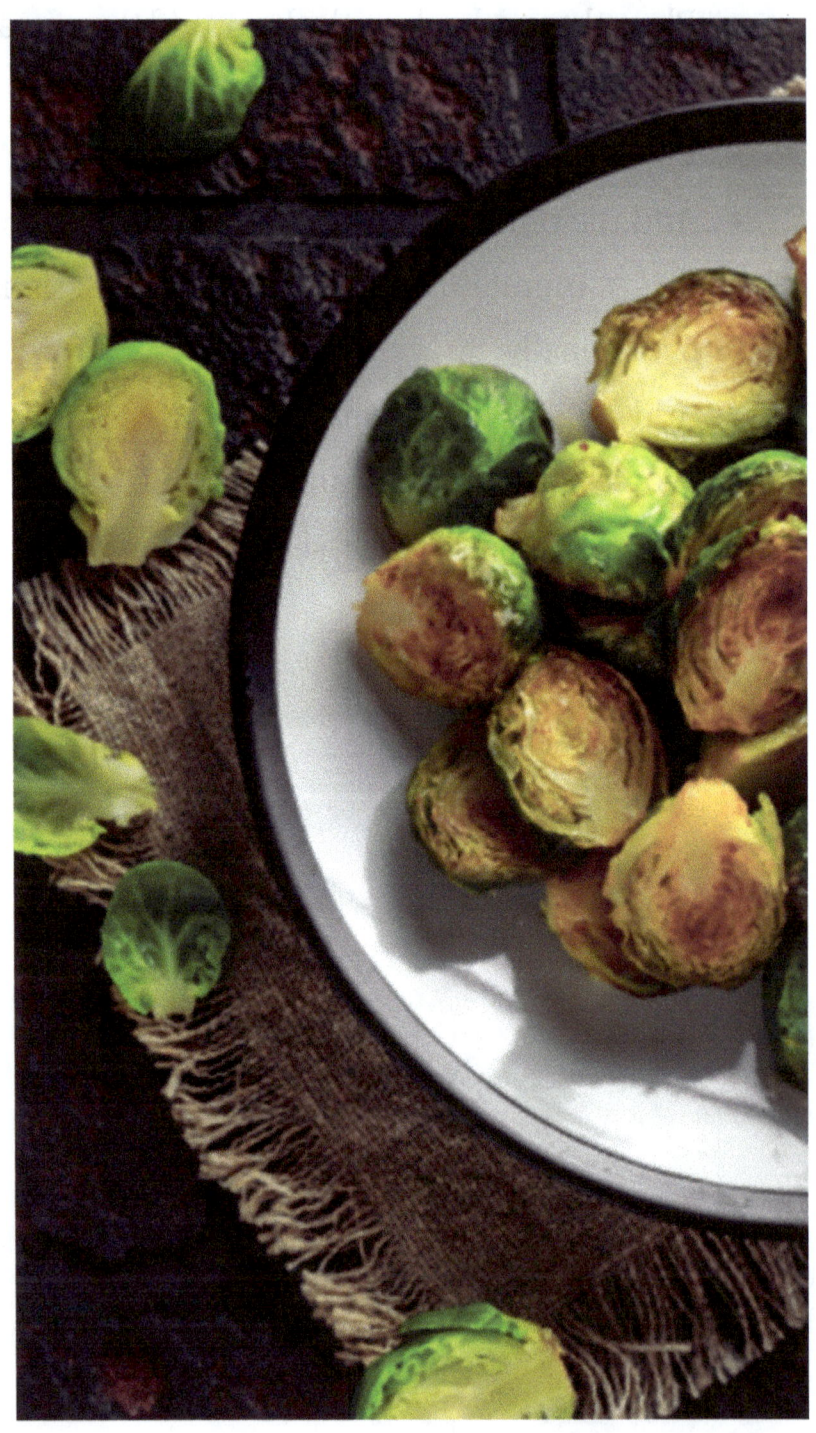

www.ingramcontent.com/pod-product-compliance
Lightning Source LLC
Chambersburg PA
CBHW070730030426
42336CB00013B/1933